CW00848199

CLINICAL NURSING POCKET BOOK

8th Edition

CLINICAL NURSING POCKET BOOK

8th Edition

Revised and updated by
Jill Gregson
Senior Education Manager
The North West London College of Nursing
and Midwifery

Mosby

Published in 1993 by Mosby–Year Book Europe Limited,
Brook House, 2–16 Torrington Place, London WC1E 7LT,
England.

First published in 1946 by Faber and Faber and titled 'A
Ward Pocket Book for the Nurse'. Sixth edition, 1965.
Reprinted 1967, 1970, 1971, 1972, 1975. Seventh edition, 1978.

Printed by BPCC Hazells Ltd, Aylesbury, England

ISBN 0 7234 18446

A CIP catalogue record for this book is available from the
British Library.

For full details of all Mosby–Year Book Europe Limited titles
please write to Mosby–Year Book Europe Limited, Brook
House, 2–16 Torrington Place, London WC1E 7LT, England.

Contents

Contents

SECTION ONE: *Ward Instruments and Equipment*

Administration of oxygen

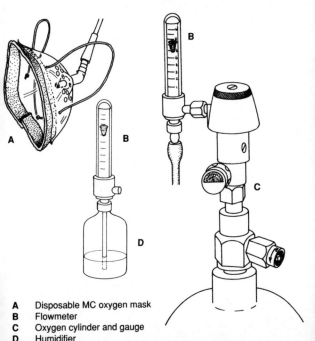

A Disposable MC oxygen mask
B Flowmeter
C Oxygen cylinder and gauge
D Humidifier

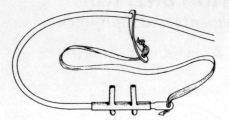

Wallace
Nasal
Cannulae

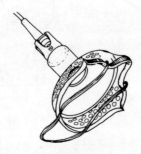

Ventimask

Ambubag

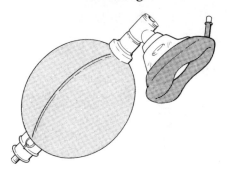

Ambubag

Airways

Guedel's airway

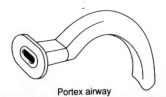

Portex airway

Cannulae

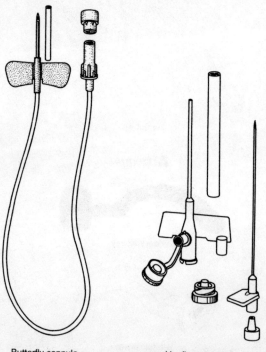

Butterfly cannula   Venflon cannula

Catheters

SECTION

A

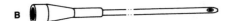

B

C

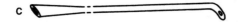

D

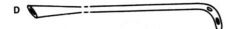

E

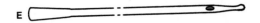

F

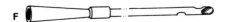

G

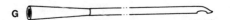

A	Foley	**E**	Olive-headed
B	Disposable Jacques	**F**	Disposable suction
C	Coudé	**G**	Rubber suction
D	Bi-Coudé		

Continuous bladder irrigation

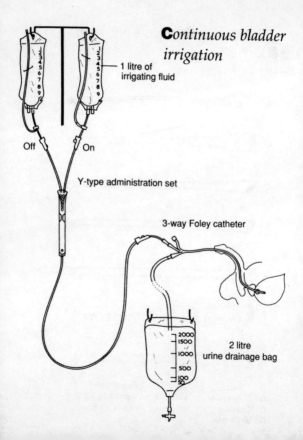

1 litre of
irrigating fluid

Off   On

Y-type administration set

3-way Foley catheter

2 litre
urine drainage bag

CVP *measurement and position of a central line*

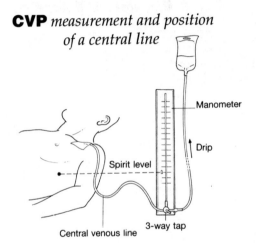

Manometer

Drip

Spirit level

Central venous line

3-way tap

Position and site for a long-term indwelling catheter

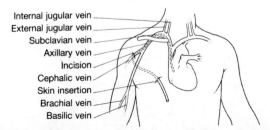

Internal jugular vein
External jugular vein
Subclavian vein
Axillary vein
Incision
Cephalic vein
Skin insertion
Brachial vein
Basilic vein

Ear, nose and throat

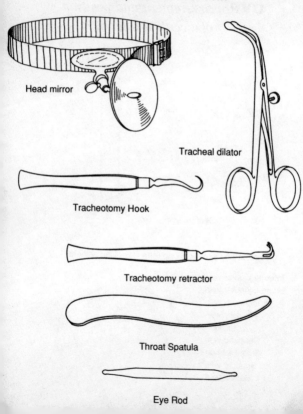

Head mirror

Tracheal dilator

Tracheotomy Hook

Tracheotomy retractor

Throat Spatula

Eye Rod

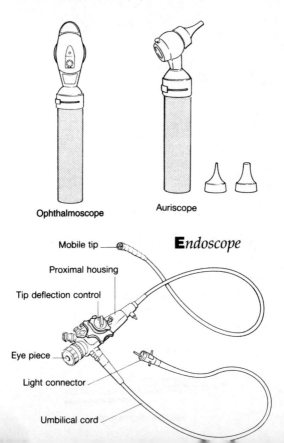

Ophthalmoscope

Auriscope

Endoscope

Mobile tip

Proximal housing

Tip deflection control

Eye piece

Light connector

Umbilical cord

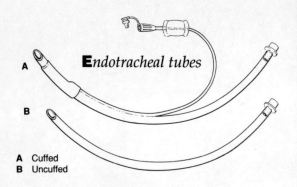

Endotracheal tubes

A Cuffed
B Uncuffed

Forceps, scalpel and clip-removers

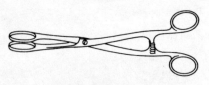

Sponge-holding forceps

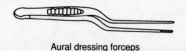

Aural dressing forceps

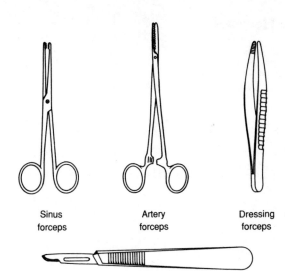

| Sinus forceps | Artery forceps | Dressing forceps |

Scalpel with Bard Parker handle and No. 15 blade

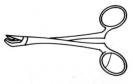

Michel-clip Remover

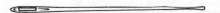

Probe

Hammers

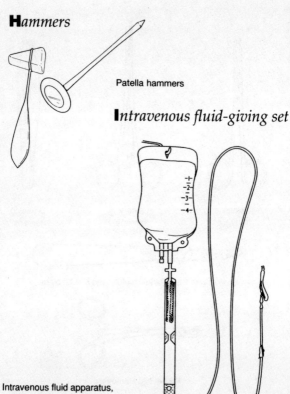

Patella hammers

Intravenous fluid-giving set

Intravenous fluid apparatus,
disposable giving set
and intravenous fluid pack

Intravenous infusion pumps

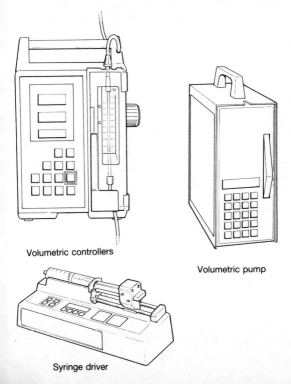

Volumetric controllers

Volumetric pump

Syringe driver

Laryngoscope

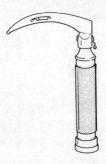

Macintosh laryngoscope

*L*umbar puncture

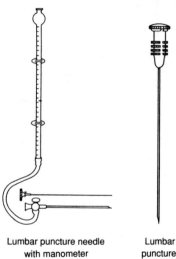

Lumbar puncture needle
with manometer

Lumbar
puncture
needle

Peritoneal dialysis apparatus

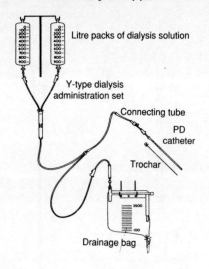

Litre packs of dialysis solution

Y-type dialysis administration set

Connecting tube

PD catheter

Trochar

Drainage bag

Protoscope

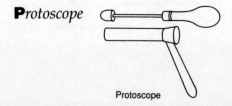

Protoscope

S*peculae*

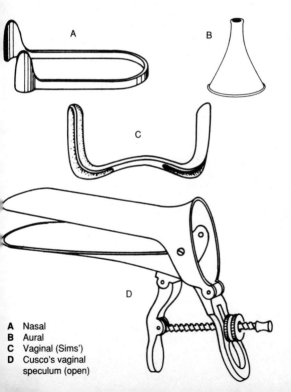

A Nasal
B Aural
C Vaginal (Sims')
D Cusco's vaginal
    speculum (open)

Sphygmomanometer

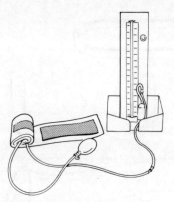

Sphygmomanometer and cuff

Syringes

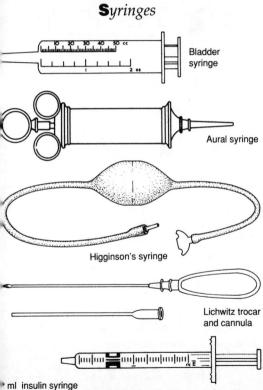

Bladder syringe

Aural syringe

Higginson's syringe

Lichwitz trocar and cannula

ml insulin syringe
insulin written on reverse side of illustration

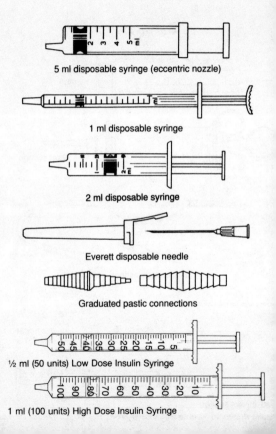

5 ml disposable syringe (eccentric nozzle)

1 ml disposable syringe

2 ml disposable syringe

Everett disposable needle

Graduated pastic connections

½ ml (50 units) Low Dose Insulin Syringe

1 ml (100 units) High Dose Insulin Syringe

Thermometers

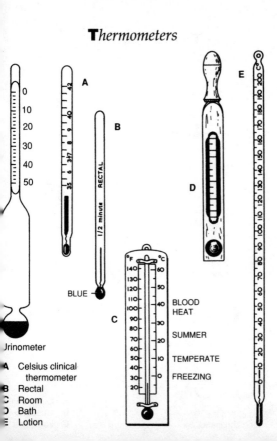

Urinometer

A Celsius clinical thermometer
B Rectal
C Room
D Bath
E Lotion

Tracheotomy tubes

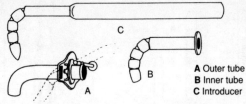

A Outer tube
B Inner tube
C Introducer

Tracheotomy tubes (Durham's Lobster-tail)

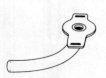

Portex tracheotomy
tube

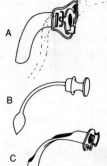

A Outer tube
B Introducer
C Inner tube

Tracheotomy tubes
(Parker's)

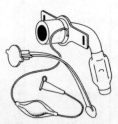

Portex cuffed tracheotomy
tube and introducer

Tubes

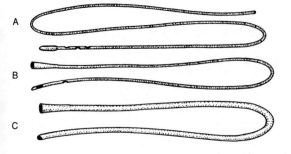

A Ryle's tube   **B** Oesophageal tube   **C** Rectal tube

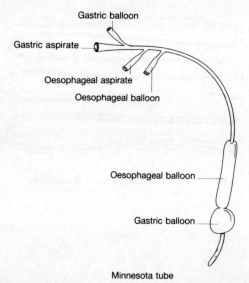

Gastric balloon

Gastric aspirate

Oesophageal aspirate

Oesophageal balloon

Oesophageal balloon

Gastric balloon

Minnesota tube

Underwater seal drain

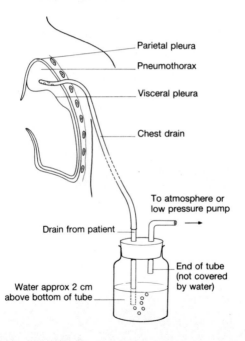

Parietal pleura

Pneumothorax

Visceral pleura

Chest drain

To atmosphere or
low pressure pump

Drain from patient

End of tube
(not covered
by water)

Water approx 2 cm
above bottom of tube

Urine drainage

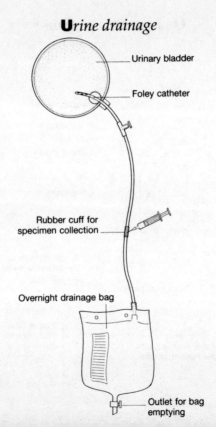

Urinary bladder

Foley catheter

Rubber cuff for
specimen collection

Overnight drainage bag

Outlet for bag
emptying

Vaginal pessaries

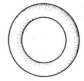

Ring pessary (PVC)

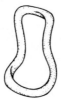

Hodge's pessary

Wound drains

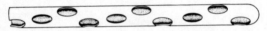

Penrose wide-bore tubing

Narrow-bore multiple perforates

Sump drain

Yeats corrugated drain

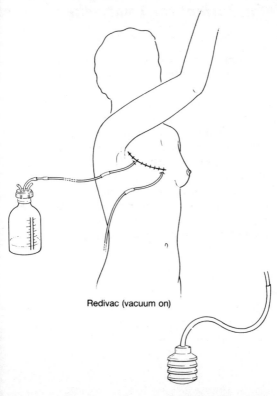

Redivac (vacuum on)

Concertina drain

SECTION TWO: *Preparation of a Patient for Treatment*

1. When preparing to give any treatment, explain to the patient what is to be done. This is important, for what seems to be a simple routine to the nurse may be alarming to the patient who is nervous and apprehensive.

2. Prepare all requirements to the last detail, so that the treatment can be done in the minimum of time and without having to leave the patient once the procedure has commenced.

3. Close the windows, screen the bed, place the patient in the correct position and cover with a blanket if the bedclothes have been turned back. Throughout the procedure, the nurse must attend to the patient's comfort and carefully observe his general condition. At all times, especially if the treatment is being performed by a doctor, the nurse should watch the reactions of the patient, noting any change in colour, pulse or respiration rate, or if he complains of nausea or faintness.

COLLECTING THE APPARATUS

1. Clean the shelves of the trolley and wash any trays to be used.
2. Collect all requirements methodically, visualizing the procedure and thinking of each item in the order in which it is to be used. This is the best way to ensure nothing is forgotten.
3. All packaging should be inspected for evidence of effective sterilization, expiry date, and any signs of damage or contamination.
4. Disposal bags for soiled dressings and used instruments should be collected.
5. The nurse's hands are to be washed before and after each treatment and dried with a paper towel.

HANDWASHING

A good hand-washing technique employed by the nurse can reduce the risk of infection to patients in hospital, and is thus most important. Studies have shown that most transient bacteria can be removed by soap and water, and resident skin flora are most effectively removed by the use of an alcoholic solution of chlorhexidine. However, additional research has demonstrated that most nurses

miss some part of their hands whilst washing,
so pay particular attention to thumbs, wrists,
under fingernails and rings, and ensure both
hands are cleansed equally thoroughly.

UNIVERSAL PRECAUTIONS

Special precautions are recommended when
treating patients known to be carrying blood-
borne viruses such as hepatitis B and H.I.V.
However, many patients will not have been
identified, and the safe approach is to assume
that any patient may be a carrier until proven
otherwise. Therefore, all blood and body fluids should be treated as infected. The risk to
staff can be reduced by the use of gloves, and
covering cuts with occlusive dressings.
Hospital policy should be followed for the
disposal of equipment, linen and body fluids,
and when caring for those with known infec-
tions.

SECTION THREE: *Methods of Sterilization and Disinfection*

Prior to disinfection or sterilization, all equipment should be thoroughly cleaned. This is usually performed by the Central Sterile Supply Service from where dressings, instruments and other apparatus are sent to the wards and departments in sterile packs.

METHODS OF DISINFECTION

Disinfection destroys vegetative pathogens and should be used only as an emergency measure.

1.   Chemical Disinfection

Hycolin 2 per cent
Hibitane 5 per cent in 70 per cent spirit
Glutaraldehyde (Cidex) 2 per cent

Immerse equipment for at least 10 minutes. Glutaraldehyde is unstable after 2 weeks and should be discarded. After chemical disinfection, items should be rinsed in sterile distilled water.

2. Heat Disinfection

Boiling. The water in the disinfector should be boiling and items placed below the level of the water line. Boil for 5 minutes.

Pasteurization. This method is used usually for endoscopes when time is not available for sterilization. The water in the pasteurization chamber is raised to 75°C and maintained for 10 minutes.

Lifting forceps may be boiled for 10 minutes and the blades placed in a container of Hibitane 5 per cent in 70 per cent spirit.

METHODS OF STERILIZATION

Sterilization destroys all micro-organisms.

1. *Autoclaves* make use of steam under pressure. With high-pressure, high-vacuum autoclaves, a pressure of 1.16 bar or 17 lb and a temperature of 120° Celcius for 20 minutes, or more commonly 2.18 bar or 32 lb pressure at a temperature of 134°C for 3½ minutes, are required for sterilization of all types of equipment.

2. *With a low-pressure and formaldehyde autoclave* the chamber is under vacuum, with a steam temperature of 70°–80°C. Formaldehyde gas is released into the steam, the amount being related to the size of the chamber. The time cycle for sterilization is 2 hours.

This method has the advantage in the sterilization of heat-labile equipment.

3. *Infra-red chambers* are used mainly for the sterilization of glass. The temperature in the chamber is raised to 180°C and maintained for 10 minutes.

4. *Ethylene oxide chambers* are used mainly for heat-labile materials such as plastic, rubber, gum elastic and endoscopes. Ten per cent ethylene oxide gas is pumped into the chamber. The sterilizing time is variable, usually 1–10 hours at a temperature of 60°C and with a high humidity content.

5. *Gamma radiation* is used by industrial suppliers of medical equipment. The radiation penetrates deeply into large cartons containing materials, so that bulk sterilization is achieved. The packaging of items of equipment where this has taken place displays a red dot to signify the fact.

SECTION FOUR:
Requirements for Unsterile Treatments and Investigations

BATHING A BABY

Baby bath
Water at 39° C
Low chair
Plastic apron
Bath towel
Thermometer
Small bowl of warm
    water
Wool swabs
Rubbish bag
Soap or bath lotion, e.g.
    Infacare

Sponge or flannel
Baby powder
Barrier cream, e.g. zinc
    and castor oil
Fine nail scissors
Safety-pins
Hair brush
Clean nappy, clean
    clothes
Clean cot linen
Dirty-linen skip

BATHING IN BED

Bath blankets
Hot and cold water
Washing bowl
Soap
Face and back flannel
Bath and hand towel
Bowl
Clean gown or pyjamas
Clean bed linen

Nail scissors or nail file
Deodorant
Talcum powder
Toothbrush and paste
Brush and comb
Glass of mouthwash
Dirty-linen container
Razor for a man

EAR SYRINGING

Towel
Tilley's forceps
2 receivers
Aural syringe
Jug lotion at 37°C
Lotion thermometer
Wool swabs
Ear buds
Treatment lamp

Auriscope
Wax hook or ringed
    probe
Warm olive oil drops
Pipette
Paper bag or receiver
Lotions, tap water or 1
    per cent sodium
    bicarbonate solution

ENEMA

Incontinence pad	*Prescribed enema*
Tray	*or*
Receiver	*Disposable phosphate*
Lubricant	*enema*
Medical wipes	*Bed pan or commode*
Jug	*Toilet roll*

Position: left lateral.

EYE DROPS INSTILLATION

Gauze squares
Prescription sheet
Drops as prescribed

Today, many eye drops are dispensed commercially in disposable plastic drop bottles.

Bottles should be discarded after 7 days and used only for the prescribed patient.

EYE IRRIGATION

Towel	Eye pad
Receiver or kidney dish	Adhesive strapping or
Gauze squares	Pad
Jug of lotion at 35°C	Bandage
Undine	Safety pin

Lotions: normal saline, sterile distilled water.

All equipment must be perfectly clean.
After eye operations, the procedure is carried
out with full aseptic precautions.

EXAMINATION OF THE EAR, NOSE AND THROAT

Treatment lamp and head mirror or head lamp and battery	Ear drops
	Nasal speculae
	Paper handkerchiefs
Auriscope	Nasal forceps
Aural speculae	Post-nasal mirror
Aural dressing forceps	Spirit lamp
Wooden applicators	Matches
Ear wool	Tongue depressors
Ring probe	Gauze squares
Tuning fork	Laryngeal mirrors
Wax hooks	Laryngoscope

Sterile swab sticks
Laboratory forms
Bowl for dentures
Mouthwash in glass
   bowl

Cocaine 10 per cent in
   throat spray
Cocaine ointment 25
   per cent
Silver nitrate sticks
Paper bag or receiver

PASSING A FLATUS TUBE

Incontinence pad
Flatus tube size 16
Medical wipes

Rectal lubricant
Bowl or paper bag

Position: left lateral.

GASTRIC LAVAGE

Trolley
Polythene sheet
Receiver
Gallipot
Medical wipes
Lubricant
Funnel
Polythene tubing
Plastic straight
   connection
Gastric tube

Large jug of water at
   37°C
1 litre jug
Pail
Vomit bowl and cloth
Bowl for dentures
Specimen bottle
Laboratory form
Mouth gag if the patient
   is unconscious

Lotions: tap water or normal saline.

N.B. If the patient is unconscious the trachea should be intubated with a cuffed tube by an anaesthetist.

WASHING HAIR IN BED

Polythene sheets
2 bath towels
Face towel
Large jug of water at 37°C
Small jug for rinsing
Sachet or bottle of shampoo
Scissors
Clean brush and comb
Hairpins, grip or rollers
Hair dryer
Protection for floor
Washing bowl

COMBING A VERMINOUS HEAD

A good light is essential
Polythene sheet
Paper bag or bowl with a lid
Toothcomb
Patient's comb
Prescribed lotion or shampoo

INCONTINENT PATIENT CARE

Inco pads
Washing bowl
Hot water
Soap
Clean drawsheet and
     bed linen

Disposable flannels
Towel
Talcum powder or pre-
     scribed ointment
Clean polythene sheet

MEDICINES ADMINISTRATION

Drug trolley contain-
ing:
Drugs and medicines
Medicine glasses
5 and 10 ml glass mea-
     sures
Teaspoons
1 ml pipettes

5 ml plastic spoons
Jug of water
Straws
Pestle and mortar
Small tray
Bowl of hot water
Prescription sheets

MOUTH CARE

Paper towel
Bowl with paper bag
Gallipots
Lotions for cleaning
    mouth, e.g. soda
    bicarbonate or gly-
    cothymol in water
Mouthwash and bowl
Bowl for dentures
Toothbrush and paste

Vaseline petroleum
    jelly
Tongue depressor
1 pair small sponge-
    holding forceps
1 pair dissecting for-
    ceps
Gauze squares or den-
    tal wipes

NASOGASTRIC INTUBATION AND FEEDING

Receiver
Tubing
Nasogastric tube of
    suitable size
Gallipots
Lubricant, water solu-
    ble, e.g. KY jelly
Medical wipes
Mouthwash
Prepared feed 37°C
50 ml syringe
Connection

5 or 10 ml syringe
Blue litmus paper
Spigot or clip
Spatula
Torch
Stethoscope
Stand and rate con-
    troller for continu-
    ous feeding
Vomit bowl and cloth
Zinc oxide strapping or
    Micropore

NEBULIZERS

Nebulizer (plus mouthpiece or mask)
Air cylinder (or electric compressor)
　　N.B. If oxygen is used, this must be prescribed
Flowmeter
Tubing
Peak flow monitor (if required)
Set flow rate to 5 litres/minute

NEUROLOGICAL EXAMINATION

Ophthalmoscope
Sphygmomanometer
Stethoscope
Patella hammer
Tuning fork
2-point discriminator
Pen torch
Laryngeal mirror
Spatulae
Gauze squares

Substances for testing
　smell and taste, e.g.
　salt, sugar, cloves,
　peppermint
Test tubes for hot and
　cold water
Pins
Cotton wool
Tape measure

OXYGEN ADMINISTRATION

Nasal route
Oxygen cylinder and key
Flowmeter
Humidifier
Green polythene tubing
Paper handkerchiefs or cotton buds in warm water
Lanolin
1 pair Wallace nasal oxygen cannulae

By Ventimask:
Correct mask to deliver prescribed percentage
Run oxygen at appropriate rate to deliver prescribed percentage
Oxygen cylinder and key
Polythene tubing
Flowmeter
Humidifier

By MC mask – *as above omitting Ventimask*
Run oxygen at 2 litres minute (MC = Mary Cantrell)

APPLICATION OF PLASTER

*Plaster bandages of
  various sizes
Stockinette
Adhesive felt
Plaster wool
Bucket of tepid water
Plaster knife
Plaster shears
Plaster benders
Plaster scissors
Polythene sheets
Polythene apron*

*Plaster boots
Dust sheets or news-
  paper
Tape measure
Skin pencil
Olive oil
Wool swabs
Materials for washing
  and shaving the
  skin may be
  required*

REMOVAL OF PLASTER

*Polythene apron
Polythene sheet
Dust sheet or news-
  papers
Plaster shears
Plaster benders
Plaster knife
Electric plaster circular
  saw*

*Plaster scissors
Container for plaster
Materials for washing
  skin
Olive oil and wool
  swabs
Sterile dressings if
  required*

PRESSURE-SORE RISK ASSESSMENT

Nursing research has established factors that indicate the level of risk for an individual patient developing pressure sores. Two of the most commonly used scoring systems are included here.

The Norton score

Designed in 1962, this scoring system was tested with patients in care-of-the-elderly settings, and is quick and simple to use.

Physical condition		*Mental condition*	
Good	4	Alert	4
Fair	3	Apathetic	3
Poor	2	Confused	2
Very bad	1	In a stupor	1

Activity		*Mobility*	
Ambulant	4	Full	4
Able to walk with help	3	Slightly limited	3
Chairbound	2	Very limited	2
Confined to bed	1	Immobile	1

Incontinence	
None	4
Occasionally	3
Usually urine	2
Doubly	1

Clinical Nursing Pocket Book

Scoring system: a score of 14 or below = at risk

Reference: Norton, D., *et al.* (1962) *An Investigation of Geriatric Problems in Hospital*: The National Corporation for the Care of Old People, London.

The Waterlow risk assessment

This is a more detailed assessment tool, developed in 1985, and can be used for patients of all ages.

Build/weight for height		Risk areas visual skin types		Sex/age	
Average	0	Healthy	0	Male	1
Above average	1	Tissue paper	1	Female	2
Obese	2	Dry	1	14–49	1
Below average	3	Oedematous	1	50–64	2
		Clammy	1	65–74	3
		Discoloured	2	75–80	4
		Broke/spot	3	81+	5

Continence		Mobility		Appetite	
Complete/ catheterized	0	Fully	0	Average	0
		Restless/ fidgety	1	Poor	1
Occasionally incontinent	1	Apathetic	2		
		Restricted	3	Nasogastric tube/fluids only	2
Cath/incontinent of faeces	2	Inert/Traction	4	NBM anorexic	3
		Chairbound	5		
Doubly incontinent	3				

Score: 10+ = at risk 15+ = high risk

SPECIAL RISKS

SPECIAL RISKS

Tissue malnutrition
e.g.

Terminal cachexia	8
Cardiac failure	5
Peripheral vascular disease	5
Anaemia	2
Smoking	1

Major surgery/trauma

Orthopaedic, below waist, spinal	5
On table >2 hours	5

Neurological deficit
e.g.

Diabetes, multiple sclerosis, paraplegia	4–6
Motor/sensory	4–6

Medication

Steroids, cytotoxics	4
Anti-inflammatory	4

Score: 20+ = very high risk

Reference: Waterlow, J. (1987) 'Calculating the risk', *Nursing Times*, 83, 39 58–60

RECORDING TEMPERATURE, PULSE AND RESPIRATION

Clinical thermometers
(each patient should
have his own ther-
mometer)
Medi-swabs
Rectal thermometers
Lubricant

Medical wipes
Paper bag for soiled
swabs
A watch with a second
hand
Charts (temperature)
Pens

RECTAL EXAMINATION

Tray
Incontinence pad
Disposable gloves
Finger stalls with cape

Medical wipes
Rectal lubricant
Proctoscope
Light

Position: left lateral.

RECTAL LAVAGE

Incontinence pad
Receiver
Rectal lubricant
Medical wipes
Rectal tube size 14
French gauge or
Charrière gauge

Tubing
Connection
Funnel
Large jug of water at
37°C
1 litre jug
Lotion thermometer

Pail
Bed pan or commode } *may be*
Toilet roll } *required*

Position: left lateral.

SHAVING

Polythene sheet   *Towel*
Tray   *Washing bowl*
Razor and blades   *Soap and flannel*
Bowl of hot water

N.B. Depilatory cream should be used to prepare areas pre-operatively. A good light is necessary.

SIGMOIDOSCOPY

Trolley   *Proctoscope and light*
Sigmoidoscope   *Battery*
Light carrier   *Bellows*
Biopsy forceps   *Light lead*
Receiver   *Specimen bottle con-*
Wool swabs   *taining formol*
Gauze squares   *saline*
Rectal lubricant   *Laboratory form*
Finger stalls with cape *Plastic apron or gown*
* or rubber gloves*   *Polythene sheet*

Position: left lateral or knee chest.

SKIN TRACTION

Polythene sheet
Materials for washing
Extension Elastoplast
Spreader or stirrup
Cord
Weights
Pulleys
Cotton and crêpe bandages
Pad of wool or sorbo
Scissors
Bed elevator

Balkan beam or Hoskin's frame
Hamilton-Russell sling }
Pillow }
Thomas splint } or
Flannel strips }
Safety-pins }
Tincture of benzoin compound in spray bottle

STEAM INHALATION

Polythene sheet
Nelson inhaler with a glass mouthpiece
Towel
Boiling water
Jug
Measure

Medication, e.g. tincture benzoin compound
Sputum carton or paper handkerchiefs
Pillow covered with a waterproof case

SUPPOSITORIES

Tray
Lubricant
Medical wipes
Glove or finger stool

Position: left lateral. Some writers suggest that if a systemic action is required then suppositories should be inserted, blunt end forward, to minimize rectal discomfort, and maximize retention. To promote defecation by local means, the pointed end should be inserted first.

TEPID SPONGING

Patient thermometer	*Face towel*
Temperature chart	*Cool drink*
Bath thermometer	*Electric fan*
Washing bowl	*Bed cradle*
Jug of water at 32°C,	*Clean bed linen*
reduce to 21°C	*Clean cotton gown*
2 to 6 sponges	*Soiled-linen container*

N.B. Reduce patient's temperature by not more than 2°C.

TO OBTAIN A THROAT SWAB

Treatment lamp and head mirror or torch
Receiver or paper bag
Tongue depressor
Sterile swabsticks
Laboratory form

N.B. Throat swabs are taken preferably in the early morning before eating.

VAGINAL EXAMINATION

Polythene sheet
2 receivers
Anglepoise lamp
Disposable polythene gloves (all sizes)
Lubricant, e.g. KY jelly
Wool swabs
Sanitary pads
Sterile swabsticks
Equipment for taking cervical smears
Laboratory forms

Sims' vaginal speculae (large, medium and small)
Cusco's vaginal speculae (large, medium and small)
Long sponge-holding forceps
Vulsellum forceps
Normal saline
Paper bags for soiled equipment

CERVICAL SMEAR (PAPANICOLAOU'S SMEAR)

Polythene sheet
Sims' vaginal speculum
Ayer's spatula
Glass slides with cover slips
Investigation form
Indelible pencil
Alcohol 95 per cent as a fixative

HIGH VAGINAL SWAB

Polythene sheet
Treatment lamp
Wool swabs
Bowl of normal saline ⎫
Cusco's vaginal speculum ⎬ *sterile*
Swabstick ⎭
Charcoal swab
Laboratory form

SECTION FIVE: *Urine Testing*

ROUTINE EXAMINATION

Note colour, smell, amount and visible deposits.
A brick-red deposit denotes the presence of urates.
A white cloudy deposit denotes the presence of phosphates or protein.

SPECIFIC GRAVITY

Place the urine in a glass deep enough to allow the urinometer to float. Stand the specimen glass on an even surface and take a reading at eye-level.
Normal specific gravity is 1010–1015.

URINE TESTING WITH TESTING STRIPS

Test for pH, protein, glucose, ketones, bilirubin and blood in the urine.

GENERAL INFORMATION

1) Multistix should be stored at a temperature of under 36°C.
2) Do not store in a refrigerator.
3) Avoid exposing to moisture, direct sunlight, heat, acid, alkali or volatile fumes.
4) Do not touch the test areas of the reagent strip.
5) Keep reagent strip away from detergents which may be found in specimen containers and on working surfaces.
6) Do not remove desiccant from bottle.
7) Replace cap of bottle immediately and tightly after removing reagent strip.
8) Read result carefully at the time specified in a good light with the test area held near the colour chart on the bottle label.
9) Do not transfer reagent strips to another bottle.
10) **Do not use strip if any test area is discoloured.**
11) Always check expiry date.

THE SPECIMEN OF URINE

Use a freshly voided, unchilled specimen only. A stale specimen gives a false reaction to some of the tests.

For quantitative tests a 24-hour specimen of urine is sent to the laboratory where a random specimen is taken and analysed.

Millistix has the added reagent for testing for the presence of urobilinogen in the urine.

DIRECTIONS FOR USE

Completely immerse all reagent areas of the strip in fresh, well-mixed, uncentrifuged urine and remove immediately, noting time. Tap the reagent stick on the edge of the urine container to remove excess urine. Compare test areas closely with the corresponding colour charts on the bottle at the time specified. Hold strip close to colour blocks and match quickly. If this instruction is not carried out carefully, faint colour development in the bilirubin reagent area may be overlooked and the test result reported as negative although bilirubin is present. If the test is negative but the presence of bilirubin is suspected retest the specimen with Ictotest reagent tablets. Note the results in the appropriate chart.

INTERPRETATIONS OF COLOUR REACTIONS

The user must bear in mind that test results with Bili-labstix are indicative rather than definite or quantitative.

pH

pH values may be interpolated to one-half unit within a range of 5–9.

Protein

A colour matching any block marked with a + sign indicates significant proteinuria.

Glucose

Light generally indicates 0.25 g per 100 ml of urine or less.
Dark indicates 0.5 g per 100 ml of urine.
Medium indicates glucose is present but does not denote amount.

Ketones

The shade of lavender or purple developed in 15 seconds indicates a small, moderate or large concentration of ketones in the specimen.

Bilirubin

The shades of brown developed at 20 seconds are read as small +, moderate ++ or large +++.

Blood

The shade of blue developed after 30 seconds indicates a small, moderate or large urinary concentration of blood (red blood cells or haemoglobin).

SECTION SIX: *Special Tests*

ESTIMATION OF BLOOD PRESSURE

Make the patient comfortable. Lift up the sleeve to clear the upper arm without it getting too tight. Abduct the arm a little way from the chest, and see that it is supported and relaxed.

Place the sphygmomanometer in a position where the mercury can easily be seen. The gauge must be vertical. Apply the cuff above the elbow with the centre of the cuff over the brachial artery, and attach to the mercury gauge. With one hand pump up the cuff and with the other feel the patient's pulse at the wrist; continue to pump until the pulse disappears.

By means of the valve allow the air to escape very gradually so that the pressure falls, watching the manometer but concentrating on the return of the pulse at the wrist. Immediately the pulse does return, read the gauge, which will give the systolic pressure in millimetres of mercury.

For an accurate estimation of both systolic and diastolic pressure repeat as before until the cuff is inflated. A stethoscope is placed on the brachial artery just below the cuff. Open the valve so that compression is gradually reduced, until the tapping sounds produced by the pulse wave are heard. Take a reading. immediately This is the systolic pressure. Continue to listen whilst the mercury falls; the sounds persist, but often change in character. Ignore these changes until they become soft and almost inaudible. Take a reading at this point, also. This is the diastolic pressure. Normal systolic pressure is approximately 100 to 140 mm Hg, and the normal diastolic 60 to 90 mm Hg (mm Hg = millimetres of mercury).

BLOOD GLUCOSE MEASUREMENT

Testing strips
Autolet, or stilette for finger prick
Paper tissues
Calibrated meter (if available)
Watch with second hand
Disposal bin for sharps
Rubbish bag
Chart

1) Prick finger.
2) Drop 1 drop of blood on the reagent strip pad.
3) Note time. Set machine.
4) Apply pressure to finger tip.
5) Remove blood by blotting with tissue for 1–2 seconds.
6) At time indicated, read result.
7) Note result on chart.

COLONOSCOPY

A colonoscope consists of a firm flexible plastic tube with a controllable end bearing a light and sometimes a camera lens, with which the entire colon can be examined. Vision is made possible by fibro-optics as in the flexible gastroscope but the colonoscope is much longer and the glass fibres are more easily damaged by bending.

Colonoscopy is used mainly for investigation purposes to detect a possible carcinoma, polyposis or ulcerative colitis, and enables multiple biopsies to be taken for histology.

In cases of a single polyp being observed diathermy can be applied.

ELECTROCARDIOGRAPH (ECG) MONITORING

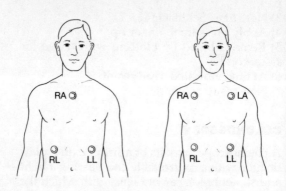

Position of chest leads

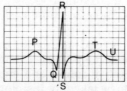

ECG for normal sinus rhythm with 60–100 beats/min.

GLUCOSE TOLERANCE TEST

The patient is given no food from 22.00 hours but may have water to drink.
The following morning:
1) The bladder is emptied. The urine is saved and a blood sample is taken.
2) The patient then drinks 75 grams of glucose dissolved in 150 to 300 ml of water.
3) A sample of blood is taken at $1/_2$, 1, $1^1/_2$ and 2 hours after the glucose has been taken.
4) Urine is collected at 1 and 2 hours.
   All specimens are labelled with the patient's name, ward, date and time of the specimen collection.

NEUROLOGICAL OBSERVATIONS

If a patient's level of consciousness is altering (or has the potential to alter), an assessment using the Glasgow Coma Scale should be undertaken. Regular observations using this scale, together with monitoring of pupillary sizes and response to light, will enable any changes to be quickly identified, and rapid action to be taken.

Glasgow Coma Scale

Eyes	Open	Spontaneously	4
		To verbal command	3
		To pain	2
	No response		1
Best motor response	To verbal command	Obeys	6
	To painful stimulus	Localizes pain	5
		Flexion-withdrawal	4
		Flexion-abnormal (decorticate rigidity)	3
		Extension (decerebrate rigidity)	2
		No response	1
Best vertebral response		Oriented and converses	5
		Disoriented and converses	4
		Inappropriate words	3
		Incomprehensible sounds	2
		No response	1
Total			**3–15**

UREA CLEARANCE TEST

The patient has a normal breakfast, but without tea or coffee. Then:
1) Completely empty the bladder and note exact time. Discard this specimen.
2) Ask the patient to drink a glass of water.
3) A specimen of blood for urea estimation is taken immediately.
4) One hour after first emptying the bladder, empty the bladder again. Label specimen 1 and note the exact time.
5) One hour later, collect another specimen of urine. Label specimen 2 and note time.
6) Send urine and blood to the laboratory.

TO SAVE A 24-HOUR SPECIMEN OF URINE

No preparation of the patient is necessary but the procedure should be explained to gain his full co-operation. Set the time to begin, e.g. at 08.00 hours.

At 08.00 hours the bladder is emptied and the urine discarded. All subsequent urine voided should be placed in the correct specimen bottle, labelled with the patient's name, age, ward, the time the collection commenced, and the appropriate date, to 08.00 hours 24 hours later (date required). At this stage, the patient should pass urine again, and this should be placed in a bottle.

Various tests require dark Winchesters, or ones containing a preservative solution. These are usually obtained from the laboratory.

SECTION SEVEN:
Requirements for Aseptic Techniques

The requirements for many of the following procedures are the same and so the details of the Basic Trolley will not be repeated every time.

Basic trolley

Sterile pack containing such items as:
Gallipots
Dressing forceps or gloves
Dressing towels ⎫
Gauze squares ⎬ sterile
Wool or foam swabs ⎭
Skin-cleaning lotion
Polythene sheet

ABDOMINAL PARACENTESIS (Tapping the abdomen)

Basic trolley
Scalpel
Robert's trocar and cannula
2 lengths of tubing   } sterile
Glass drip connection
Drainage bag

Many-tailed bandage   Gloves
Safety-pins   Specimen bottle
Adhesive strapping   Laboratory form
Gate clip   Fluid chart
Face masks

N.B. The patient must empty his bladder. Catheterization may be necessary.

ANTRUM PUNCTURE AND WASHOUT

Shoulder cape   Lotion thermometer
Receiver for soiled   Lifting forceps (sterile)
   instruments   2 specimen bottles
Lamp and head mirror   Laboratory form
Cocaine ointment 25   Bowl 14 cm
   per cent   Paper handkerchiefs

Mouthwash
2 nasal speculae
Lichtwitz' trocar and cannulae
Antral syringe or Higginson's syringe

Jug containing normal saline 37°C
Cotton-wool balls
Wooden applicators
20 ml syringe
Local anaesthetic

ASPIRATION OF A PNEUMOTHORAX AND CHEST DRAINAGE

Basic trolley
2 sterile pneumothorax needles
Tape
Local anaesthetic
Scalpel

Suture materials
Dressing
Clamps
Gloves
Sedative cough linctus
Prescription sheet

Position: either lateral, exposing affected side, a pillow under the chest and the arm extended above the head; or leaning forward over a bed table.

A thoracotomy drain and underwater seal drainage bottle may be used for this procedure, in which case a Robert's suction apparatus will be required.

BLADDER IRRIGATION

This can be performed in two ways:
1. By a bladder syringe – useful when bladder antiseptics have been prescribed.
2. By continuous closed irrigation (*see* page 16).

Catheter in situ
Receiver
Bladder syringe
Measuring jug
Irrigating fluid at 37°C } *sterile*
Large bowl or pail
Polythene sheet
Lotion thermometer

Lotion: sterile distilled water or sterile normal saline.

BLOOD GROUPING

International Classification
Provided the Rhesus factor is compatible:
Group A can receive from Group AO.
Group B can receive from Group BO.
Group AB. Universal recipient.
Group O. Universal donor, can receive only from Group O.

BLOOD TRANSFUSION OR INTRA-VENOUS INFUSION

Basic trolley
Butterfly cannulae
    0.6 mm or size 23
    0.8 mm or size 21 } *sterile*
    1.1 mm or size 19   *(mm = millimetre)*

Venflon cannulae
Sterile intravenous
    giving set (with fil-
    ters if blood or blood
    products are to be
    administered)
Sphygmomanometer or
    tourniquet
Intravenous stand
Splint
Bandage and safety-pin

Adhesive strapping
Pillow with protective
    cover
Bag or bottle of normal
    saline, glucose 5 per
    cent, blood or other
    solution for infusion
Temperature, pulse
    and respiration
    chart if blood is
    given

It may be necessary to cut down onto a vein; therefore, the following equipment should be available. This may be provided in a cut-down pack.

Scalpel
2 pairs fine-toothed dissecting forceps
2 pairs small artery forceps
1 pair small scissors
1 aneurysm needle   } *sterile*
Small curved cutting needle
Fine plain catgut
Nylon sutures
Face masks
Rubber gloves

FEMALE CATHETERIZATION

A good light is essential
Polythene sheet
Receiver for soiled swabs
Warm antiseptic solution
Sterile lubricant, e.g. KY jelly
Dressing towel
Wool swabs
Bowl
Gauze squares to apply lubricant to   } *sterile*
*   catheters*
Jacques catheters size 12–16
2 dressing forceps
Receiver

Normal saline
Chlorhexidine
Sterile disposable
 gloves
Sterile anaesthetic gel

Lifting forceps
Measuring jug
Specimen bottle
Laboratory form

Position: dorsal with knees flexed and abducted.

See Foley catheter (page 36) for continuous bladder drainage.

MALE CATHETERIZATION

A good light is essential
Polythene sheets
Receiver for soiled
 swabs
Measuring jug
Specimen bottle

Laboratory form
Anaesthetic gel, e.g.
 Lignocaine
 hydrochloride
 2 per cent in a sterile lubricant basis
Warm antiseptic lotion

Dressing towels
Bowl
Wool swabs
Gauze squares
Catheters, several sizes
Nozzle for lubricant
Receiver

} sterile

For use with a Foley catheter (continuous bladder drainage):

10 ml syringe
Water $\left.\right\}$ *sterile*
Catheter drainage bag
Drainage bag stand
Adhesive strapping
Safety-pin

CENTRAL VENOUS PRESSURE LINE

Basic trolley
Bard Parker handle Number 15 blade
Bard–I–Cath 12 inches intravenous catheter
Intravenous giving set
Intravenous stand
Central venous pressure manometer set
Manometer
Fluid balance chart
Central venous pressure chart

N.B. The venous pressure is read as millimetre of water.
The subclavian veins are the most commonly used.

CHEST ASPIRATION

Basic trolley
50 ml syringe
Chest aspirating needles
of various lengths and size } *sterile*
2-way tap
Rubber tubing and sinker
Measuring jug

Specimen bottle	*Medicine glass*
Laboratory form	*Prescription sheet*
Sputum cup or paper	*Adhesive dressing or*
handkerchiefs	*collodion flex*
Sedative cough medi-	*Face masks*
cine, e.g. linctus	*Gloves*
codeine	

Position: sitting up leaning forward over a bed-table or supported in the lateral position. Patient's X-rays should be available.

INTRAMUSCULAR INJECTION

Tray
Medi-swabs (if used)
Sterile syringes of appropriate size: 1, 2 or 5 ml
Selection of sterile needles
Drug prescribed
Prescription sheet

N.B. Not more than 4 ml should be injected into one site. Needle should be inserted at 90 degree angle.

Sites For Intramuscular Injection

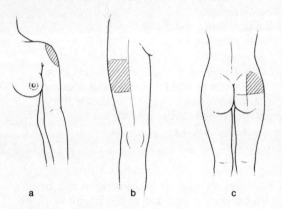

a   b   c

(a) Outer aspect of shoulder
(b) Antero-lateral aspect of the thigh
(c) Upper and outer quadrant of the buttock

SUBCUTANEOUS INJECTION

Equipment as for intramuscular injection
Syringe
Needle

N.B. Needle should be inserted at 45 degree angle.

LUMBAR PUNCTURE

Basic trolley	*3 sterile specimen*
2 sterile lumbar punc-	*bottles and 1 glucose*
ture needles	*specimen bottle*
Sterile manometer,	*Laboratory form*
tubing and connec-	*2 per cent liq. iodine*
tion	*Adhesive dressing*
	Gloves

Position: the patient should be lying on a firm surface in the left lateral position, with the knees drawn up under the chin.

PERITONEAL DIALYSIS

Basic trolley
Lifting forceps
Bard Parker handle and a No. 11 blade
Hypodermic needles Nos. 1 and 25
Peritoneal dialysis catheter
  'Trocath' 12 inches
Y-type peritoneal giving set
Peritoneal dialysis drainage bag   } sterile
Curved cutting needle
Needle holder
Nylon suture
Scissors
Gloves
3 extra cotton towels

Intravenous stand	Label for additives to
Lignocaine	dialysate
Dialysis fluid	Elastoplast
Dialysis sheet	Warming chamber for
Heparin	dialysate
Potassium	Bed cradle
2 ml syringe	
No. 1 needle	

N.B. If not anuric the patient must empty his bladder.

TRACHEOTOMY

Basic trolley
1 scalpel
4 pairs artery forceps
2 pairs toothed dissecting forceps
1 pair scissors
2 double hooked retractors
1 blunt hook
1 sharp hook
Tracheal dilators
Tracheotomy tubes of various types
   and size
Suction catheters
Curved cutting needles
Nylon skin sutures
Fine plain catgut
Needle holder
} *sterile*

Suction apparatus   *Sandbag*
Face masks   *Tape for tracheotomy*
Gauze   *tubes*
Sterile gloves   *A very good light*

CARE OF TRACHEOTOMY

Polythene sheet	*Spare tapes*
Soda bicarbonate solu-	*Paper handkerchiefs*
tion	*Suction apparatus*
Tracheotomy tube, brush	*Bowl of sterile water for*
or pipe cleaners	*cleaning catheters*
Gauze	*after use with suction*

Foam dressings
Suction catheters
Spare tracheotomy tubes the same size ⎫
as the one in situ ⎬ *sterile*
Tracheal dilators ⎪
2 pairs dressing forceps ⎭
Disposable polythene gloves

N.B. Writing paper, pencil, mirror and bell
will be required by the patient.

CLEAN SPECIMEN OF URINE—FEMALE

Bowl of warm antiseptic lotion ⎫
Wool swabs ⎬ *sterile*
Measuring jug ⎭
Specimen bottle
Laboratory form
Bed pan and cover
Soap and flannel .
Towel

MID-STREAM SPECIMEN OF URINE— MALE

Soap and water, saline or a solution that does not contain disinfectant

Wool swabs
Measuring jug   }   sterile
Funnel
Specimen bottle
Laboratory form
Urinal

WOUND DRAINAGE

Wounds can be drained by gravity, capillary action or pressure. The objective may be to initiate the discharge of pus, to prevent the accumulation of fluid post-surgery, to prevent surface healing over a deep infected wound, or to provide a means of irrigation if the wound is heavily contaminated.

Drains can be open into a dressing, or drainage bag – gauze wick or corrugated plastic, or a hollow tube, cut to the appropriate size.

Closed drains are part of an integrated system – drain, connecting tubing and collection container – and are usually made of plastic.

WOUND DRESSINGS

A wide variety of dressings is now available and each has a different function for a particular type of wound. It is important to use the correct type of dressing, and therefore specialist advice or literature should be consulted before a dressing is used. The following is provided as an introduction only, and further reading is recommended.

Hydrocolloid dressings (solid particles dispersed in liquid)

When placed on the surface of an exuding wound, the dressing absorbs liquid and forms a gel. Most are backed with a continuous plastic film, thus preventing organisms from the external environment reaching the surface of the wound. They are relatively easy to use on wounds such as leg ulcers, and pressure sores. They should not be used on clinically infected wounds.

Semi-permeable film dressings

These should overlap the wound by 3–4 cm and be used on abrasions, minor burns, donor sites, or superficial pressure sores. They allow the skin to breathe, and prevent the build-up of water vapour, allowing the wound to be observed. They should not be used on heavy exuding wounds, or infected or deep wounds.

Absorbent dressings

These are designed to remove exudate and the results of infection. Non-adherent types are now available but they can stick to the wound, causing pain as they are removed.

SIMPLE DRESSING

Polythene sheet if necessary
Bag for soiled instruments
Lifting forceps
Adhesive strapping, Micropore or Elastoplast
2 gallipots ⎫
2 receivers ⎪
4 pairs dressing forceps or gloves ⎬ *sterile*
Dressing towel ⎪
Dressings ⎭
Bag for soiled dressings
Bandages
Safety-pins
Skin-cleaning lotions
Hand towel

OPENING AN ABSCESS

As for a simple dressing.
In addition:
1 sinus forceps
1 silver probe
1 Volkmann's spoon } *sterile*
Scalpel
1 pair scissors
Rubber and gauze drains } *sterile*
Safety-pins
Rubber gloves
Gown and mask
Swabstick
Stuart's medium
Laboratory form
Local analgesia may be given but more often a
*   general anaesthetic*
Consent form

SUTURING A WOUND

A basic trolley   *Curved cutting needles*
Scissors   *Nylon suture*
1 pair toothed dissect-   *Local anaesthetic*
*   ing forceps*   *Sterile syringe*
Needle holder   *Sterile needles*

Scalpel
Probe
Sinus forceps
2 pair artery forceps ⎫ *these may be*
Rubber and gauze ⎬ *required for other*
　drains ⎭ *than clean stitched*
Safety-pins 　　　 *wounds*
Catgut
Rubber gloves

N.B. A general anaesthetic may be given, in which case a consent form will be required.

Removal of sutures

As for a simple dressing.
In addition:
Stitch scissors or stitch cutter

Removal of clips

As for a simple dressing.
In addition:
1 pair Michel clip removers or a pair of artery
　forceps for butterfly clips

SECTION EIGHT:
Weights and Measures

METRIC MEASURES IN SI UNITS

SI units = *Système International d'Unités*, or International System of Units

Common symbols and conversion factors

1 g	=	0.035 of an ounce
1 kg	=	2.2 pounds
1 oz	=	28.35 grams
1 lb	=	453.6 grams
1 st	=	6.35 kilograms

1 microgram (μg)	=	0.000 001 gram
1 milligram (mg)	=	0.001 gram
1 centigram	=	0.01 gram
1 gram (g or G)	=	1.0 gram
1 decagram	=	10.0 gram
1 hectogram	=	100.0 gram
1 kilogram (Kg)	=	1,000.0 gram

MOLECULAR UNITS

Mol	=	mole—for molecular substances, this is the molecular weight in grams		
mmol	=	millimole	=	0.001 of a mole
μ mol	=	micromole	=	0.000 001 of a mole
n mol	=	nanomole	=	0.000 000 001 of a mole

LENGTH

μm	=	micrometre	=	0.000001 of a metre
mm	=	millimetre	=	0.001 of a metre
cm	=	centimetre	=	0.01 of a metre
m	=	metre	=	1.0 metre

25.4 mm	=	1 inch
2.54 cm	=	1 inch
0.30 m	=	1 foot
0.91 m	=	1 yard

The symbol S should not be added to make plurals. In SI units S = seconds.

PRESSURE

The unit of pressure is a pascal. These units are not yet in general use.

µPa	=	micropascal	=	0.000 001 of a pascal
mPa	=	millipascal	=	0.001 of a pascal
kPa	=	kilopascal	=	1.0 pascal
MPa	=	megapascal	=	1 000 000 pascal
GPa	=	gigapascal	=	1 000 000 000 pascal

This unit should be used in place of measuring mm Hg in measuring blood pressure.

1 mm Hg	=	133.3 Pa
150 mm Hg	=	20 kilopascal
Hg	=	mercury

THERMOMETRIC EQUIVALENTS

Celsius		Fahrenheit
35.0°	=	95.0°
36.2°	=	97.2°
36.8°	=	98.2°
37.8°	=	100.0°
38.4°	=	101.0°
39.0°	=	102.2°
39.8°	=	103.6°
40.2°	=	104.4°
41.0°	=	105.8°

To convert °F to °C subtract 32, and multiply by $5/9$, e.g. $101°F - 32 = 69 \times 5/9 = 38.3°C$.

To convert °C to °F multiply by $9/5$ and then add 32, e.g. 37°C $\times 9/5 = 66.6 + 32 = 98.6$°F.

TIME

24-hour clock
   1 AM–12 MD as usual
   1 PM–12 MN = 13.00 hr–24.00 hr

VOLUME

ml	=	millilitre	=	0.001 of a litre
cl	=	centilitre	=	0.01 of a litre
dl	=	decilitre	=	0.1 of a litre
L	=	litre	=	1.0 litre

1 fluid ounce	=	28.4 ml
1 pint	=	568.0 ml

SECTION NINE:
Drug Dosage Calculations

CALCULATING THE CORRECT DOSE

The formula for calculating doses is:

$$\frac{\text{dose prescribed}}{\text{dose available}} \times \text{volume available}$$

Example
Dose prescribed: diazepam 2 mg; dose available: diazepam 10 mg in 2 ml

$$\frac{2}{10} \times 2 = \frac{4}{10} = 0.4 \text{ml}$$

INTRAVENOUS THERAPY: CALCULATING THE DRIP RATE

The formula is:

$$\frac{\text{prescribed volume (ml)}}{\text{prescribed time (hours)}} \times \frac{\text{drops per ml}}{60}$$

A regular giving set will normally deliver 20 drops per ml of clear fluids, or 15 drops per ml of blood. Microgiving sets deliver 60 drops per ml of clear fluids. Always check the manufacturer's instructions on the pack.

Example
Prescribed: 1 litre normal saline in 8 hours.

$$\frac{1000}{8} \times \frac{20}{60} = \frac{2000}{48} = 41.7$$

Therefore, deliver approximately 42 drops per minute.

SECTION TEN:
Misuse of Drugs Act 1971

Lists the drugs to be controlled and classifies them for the purposes of the Act.
Regulations made under this Act restrict the use of habit-forming drugs. Included are:

Amphetamines
Cocaine
Codeine for injection
Dexamphetamine
Dextromoramide   (Palfium)
Diamorphine
Diconal
Dihydrocodeine injection   (D.F. 118)
Fentanyl
Leverphanol   (Dromoran)
Methadone
Methaqualone   (in Mandrax)
Methylamphetamine
Methylphenidate   (Ritalin)
Morphine

Nepenthe
Pamergan preparations
Papaveretum   (Omnopon)
Pethidine
Phenazocine   (Narphen)
Phenmetrazine   (Preludin)
Phenoperidine

SECTION ELEVEN:
Poisons Act 1972

The poison rules made under this act control the supply and sale of poisonous substances. Among the drugs included in the various Schedule of Rules are:

Alkaloids and their salts including:

Antihistamines
Atropine
Barbituric acid, its salts and derivatives
Codeine
Digitalis glycosides
Dihydrocodeine D.F. 118 ORAL
Emetine
Ephedrine
Ergometrine
Ergotamine
Hyoscine
Insulin
Most of the tranquillizers and anti-depressants
Strychnine
Sulphonamides

Many of the drugs included are available on prescription only. The preparation and supply of antibiotics, corticosteroids, and other biological preparations are controlled by the Medicines Act part III.

SECTION TWELVE:
Food Values

UNITS OF ENERGY

Unit   1 kilocalorie   unit of energy

The Calorie or kilocalorie used in nutrition is the amount of heat required to raise the temperature of 1,000 grams of water 1 degree Celsius, e.g. 15°C to 16°C.

The word calorie used in nutrition should be written with a capital C.

Energy value   Unit   1 Joule   Metric

The unit of energy is the kilojoule. It is the amount of energy expended when 1 kilogram is moved 1 metre by a force of 1 Newton.

A Newton is the force applied to a mass of 1 kilogram, giving it an acceleration of 1 metre per second squared.

ENERGY YIELD

1 gram protein	=	4.1 kilocalorie
		17.1544 kilojoule
1 gram carbohydrate	=	3.75 kilocalorie
		15.69 kilojoule
1 gram fat	=	9.3 kilocalorie
		38.9112 kilojoule

1 kilocalorie = 4.184 kilojoule. To convert 1 kilocalorie to kilojoule multiply the number of Calories by 4.184.

1 000 joule	=	1 kilojoule
1 000 000 joule	=	1 megajoule

DAILY ENERGY REQUIREMENTS

Average	
man	3,000 kcal or 12.6 megajoule
Average	
woman	2,200 kcal or 9.2 megajoule
Pregnant	
woman	2,400 kcal or 10.0 megajoule
Nursing	
mother	2,700 kcal or 11.0 megajoule
Boy aged	
12 to 15 years	2,800 kcal or 11.7 megajoule

Girl aged	
12 to 15 years	2,300 kcal or 9.6 megajoule
Boy aged	
15 to 18 years	3,000 kcal or 12.6 megajoule
Girl aged	
15 to 18 years	2,300 kcal or 9.6 megajoule
Patient in bed	1,800 to 2,000 or 7.35 to 8.40
Baby	110 kcal to 120 kcal per kilo of body weight = 4.60 kjoule to 5.02 kjoule per kilo of body weight

ENERGY VALUES OF SOME FOODS

Composition per ounce or 28.35 gram

Cow's milk	18 kcalorie or 77 kjoule
Sugar	112 kcalorie or 469 kjoule
Single cream	54 kcalorie or 225 kjoule
White bread	253 kcalorie or 1,060 kjoule
Butter	211 kcalorie or 884 kjoule
Average egg	45 kcalorie or 188 kjoule
Cheddar cheese	117 kcalorie or 490 kjoule
Cottage cheese	32 kcalorie or 137 kjoule
Cooked lean beef	89 kcalorie or 373 kjoule
Cooked chicken	52 kcalorie or 219 kjoule
White fish	19 kcalorie or 82 kjoule
Potato boiled	23 kcalorie or 94 kjoule

NUTRITIONAL CONTENT

Some foods rich in:

Protein	meat, fish, eggs, cheese, soya beans and nuts, milk.
Carbohydrate	sugar, cereals, potatoes, bread, flour and dried fruits.
Fat	butter, cream, cheese, eggs, and vegetable oils.
Calcium	cheese, egg yolk, milk, carrots, cabbage, ice cream.
Phosphorus	cheese, egg yolk, mackerel, halibut, cod, and liver.
Potassium	prunes, potatoes (raw), sprouts, liver, milk, eggs, cheddar cheese, bacon.
Iron	liver, kidney, eggs, beef, cocoa, wholemeal bread, and dried apricots.
Vitamin A	carrots, halibut liver oil, cod liver oil, liver, butter, cheese, eggs and milk.
Vitamin B	yeast, Marmite, Bemax, wholemeal bread, peanuts and egg yolk.
Vitamin C	Citrus fruits, watercress, sprouts and cabbage.
Vitamin D	cod liver oil, halibut liver oil, herrings, milk, cheese, butter, milk and eggs.
Vitamin E	wheat germ, meat and eggs.
Vitamin K	liver.

SECTION THIRTEEN:
Laboratory Normal Values

BLOOD NORMAL VALUES

Albumin	40–50 g/L
Alkaline phosphatase	30–130 units/L
Bilirubin (total)	5–7 mol/L
Calcium	2.1–2.6 mmol/L
pCO_2	4.7–6.0 kPa
Chloride	100–10^6 mmol/L
Clotting time	< 15 minutes
Creatinine	62–132 mmol/L
Erythrocyte sedimentation rate	1–13 mm/hr
Glucose	3.9–5.6 mmol/L
Haematocrit	42–50%
Haemoglobin	13–16 g/100 ml
Iron	9.0–26.9 mmol/L
Magnesium	0.8–1.3 mmol/L
Mean corpuscular volume	80–94 fL
Osmolality	280–295 mmol/kg
Oxygen saturation	96–100 per cent
pH	7.35–7.45
Phosphatase (acid)	36–175 nmols^{-1}/L

Phosphatase (alkaline)	0.18–0.4 nmols^{-1}/L
Platelet count	200–350 × 10^6/L
pO$_2$	10.0–13.3 kPa
Potassium	3.5–5.0 mmol/L
Sodium	135–145 mmol/L
Urea	2.5–6.6 mmol/L
White cell count	4.0–10.0 × 10^6/litre

CEREBROSPINAL FLUID (CSF) NORMAL VALUES

Pressure	8–18 cm of water
Chloride	120–130 mmol/L
Glucose	2.8–4.2 mmol/L
Protein	0.15–0.45 g/L
Cell count	0–5

SECTION FOURTEEN:
Incubation Periods of Infectious Diseases

Disease	Incubation period	Period of isolation
Chickenpox (varicella)	7–23 days	Until last scab has separated
Diphtheria	1–6 days	Until 3 consecutive nose and throat swabs are negative
German measles (rubella)	17–18 days	Seven days from appearance of rash
Influenza	1–3 days	Up to 7 days
Measles (morbilli)	10–14 days	Fourteen days from appearance of rash
Meningococcal meningitis	2–10 days	Twenty-four hours after therapy commences
Mumps (infective parotitis)	7–23 days	One week after swelling has subsided
Poliomyelitis	7–14 days	Usually 3 weeks
Salmonella	6–48 hours	Until 3 consecutive stools are negative
Viral hepatitis (A)	15–50 days	First 2 weeks from onset
Viral hepatitis (B)	45–180 days	Isolate blood and body fluids until negative
Whooping cough (pertussis)	7–14 days	Three to 4 weeks

SECTION FIFTEEN:
Common Abbreviations

a.c.	*ante cibos*	before meals
ad lib	*ad libitum* ·	to the desired amount
a a	*ana*	of each
aq. dest.	*aqua destillata*	distilled water
b.d.	*bis die*	twice a day
caps.		capsules
cat.	*cataplasma*	a poultice
c.c.	*cum cibis*	with food
comp.	*compositus*	compounded of
elix.		elixir
gutt.	*gutta or guttae*	drop or drops
i.m.		intramuscular
inf.	*infusum*	an infusion
inj.	*injectio*	an injection
i.v.		intravenous
n.b.m.		nil by mouth
p.r.	*per rectum*	by the rectum
p.r.n.	*pro re nata*	as occasion arises
p.v.	*per vaginam*	by the vagina
q.d.	*quater in die*	four times a day

q.h.	*quater horis*	four hourly
R	*recipe*	take
stat.	*statim*	immediately
t.d.s.	*ter in die*	let it be taken
	sumendum	three
		times a day
ung.	*unguentum*	ointment

SECTION SIXTEEN: *Code of Professional Conduct for the Nurse, Midwife and Health Visitor (1992)*

Each registered nurse, midwife and health visitor shall act, at all times, in such a manner as to:

- safeguard and promote the interests of individual patients and clients;
- serve the interests of society;
- justify public trust and confidence and
- uphold and enhance the good standing and reputation of the professions.

As a registered nurse, midwife or health visitor, you are personally accountable for your practice and, in the exercise of your professional accountability, must:

1 act always in such a manner as to promote and safeguard the interests and well-being of patient and clients;

2 ensure that no action or omission on your part, or within your sphere of responsibility, is detrimental to the interests, condition or safety of patients and clients;

3 maintain and improve your professional knowledge and competence;

4 acknowledge any limitations in your knowledge and competence and decline any duties or responsibilities unless able to perform them in a safe and skilled manner;

5 work in an open and co-operative manner with patients, clients and their families, foster their independence and recognise and respect their involvement in the planning and delivery of care;

6 work in a collaborative and co-operative manner with health care professionals and others involved in providing care, and recognise and respect their particular contributions within the care team;

7 recognise and respect the uniqueness and dignity of each patient and client, and respond to their need for care, irrespective of their ethnic origin, religious beliefs, personal attributes, the nature of their health problems or any other factor;

8 report to an appropriate person or authority, at the earliest possible time, any conscientious objection which may be relevant to your professional practice;

9 avoid any abuse of your privileged relationship with patients and clients and of the privileged access allowed to their person, property, residence or workplace;

10 protect all confidential information concerning patients and clients obtained in the course of professional practice and make disclosures only with consent, where required by the order of a court or where you can justify disclosure in the wider public interest;

11 report to an appropriate person or authority, having regard to the physical, psychological and social effects on patients and clients, any circumstances in the environment of care which could jeopardise standards of practice;

12 report to an appropriate person or authority any circumstances in which safe and appropriate care for patients and clients cannot be provided;

13 report to an appropriate person or authority where it appears that the health or safety

of colleagues is at risk, as such circumstances may compromise standards of practice and care;

14 assist professional colleagues, in the context of your own knowledge, experience and sphere of responsibility, to develop their professional competence, and assist others in the care team, including informal carers, to contribute safely and to a degree appropriate to their roles;

15 refuse any gift, favour or hospitality from patients or clients currently in your care which might be interpreted as seeking to exert influence to obtain preferential consideration and

16 ensure that your registration status is not used in the promotion of commercial products or services, declare any financial or other interests in relevant organisations providing such goods or services and ensure that your professional judgement is not influenced by any commercial considerations.

Reproduced with the kind permission of the UKCC.

SECTION SEVENTEEN:
Useful Phone and Bleep Numbers

Area   **Phone number**

Switchboard

Cardiac Arrest

Fire

Security

Pharmacy

Dietician

Physiotherapist

X-Ray

Outpatients

Index